Renata Dalberto
Viviane Koepp
Geisson Marcos Nardi

Profile of nursing graduates in the world of work:

Renata Dalberto
Viviane Koepp
Geisson Marcos Nardi

Profile of nursing graduates in the world of work:

From training, to professional performance

ScienciaScripts

Cover image: www.ingimage.com

This book is a translation from the original published under ISBN 978-613-9-62369-3.

Publisher:
Sciencia Scripts
is a trademark of
Dodo Books Indian Ocean Ltd. and OmniScriptum S.R.L publishing group

120 High Road, East Finchley, London, N2 9ED, United Kingdom
Str. Armeneasca 28/1, office 1, Chisinau MD-2012, Republic of Moldova, Europe
Printed at: see last page
ISBN: 978-620-7-72422-2

SUMMARY

ACKNOWLEDGMENTS

I thank God, who gave me life, for all the doors he *has* opened in my path and for every opportunity he has given me.

I would like to thank a very special person, the most important person in this achievement, without whom this moment would not have come true, a determined, hard-working person, who proved today that it is worth dreaming and never giving up, because dreams do come true, you just have to want them to. That person is ME!

To my parents, for their unconditional support at every moment of my life, to whom I dedicate every victory.

To my husband Fabiano, for his support and understanding.

To my brothers, for their encouragement.

To my advisor, Viviane Kopp Nardi, for her guidance.

To my co-supervisor Geisson Marcos Nardi, for his teachings and guidance.

To the coordinator of the Nursing Course, Fabiana Meneguetti Dallacosta, for the alternatives and opportunities she made available for this moment to materialize and for her guidance.

To the course lecturers, for their teaching, support, understanding and knowledge during this journey.

To the nursing graduates, for also taking the time to contribute to this study.

There is so much more to thank... to all those who, although not named, have given me their invaluable support at all times and with their affectionate presence, my sincere and affectionate thanks!

"Nursing is an art; and to carry it out as an art, it requires a devotion as exclusive, a preparation as rigorous, as the work of any painter or sculptor; for what is it to treat the dead canvas or the cold marble compared to treating the living body, the temple of God's spirit? It is one of the arts; one could say, the most beautiful of the arts!"

Florence Nightingale

SUMMARY

The world of work is undergoing changes in all areas. Globalization and technological advances have made the world of work more demanding, so young people need to be trained to enter the job market. The aim of this study was to characterize the profile and difficulties encountered by nurses in the academic-professional transition at a university located in the Midwest of Santa Catarina. This is a quantitative-qualitative study. Data was collected between June and July 2016 using a semi-structured questionnaire via Google Docs. A total of 74 graduates of the Nursing course took part, having graduated between 2009 and 2015. The results show that the majority of graduates had no difficulty getting their first job, and entered the world of work by various means. They reported criticisms of the course, such as a hospital-centered view, a low number of hours of practical classes and a lack of experience on the part of the teachers, especially in the field of internships, as well as pointing out the need for improvements. It was concluded that the majority of graduates are in the world of work and that the course offers them the conditions to compete professionally, but that they should be aware of market needs and trends.

Keywords: Nursing. Nursing education. Labor market.

1 INTRODUCTION

The world of work is undergoing changes in all areas. Globalization and technological advances have made the market more demanding when it comes to hiring new employees, so young people need to train to keep up with the changes and enter the workforce. For Silva, Oliveira and Oliveira (2015, p. 40), the labor market "[...] can be understood as a mechanism of supply and demand constituted by companies, opportunities and the process of attracting a set of candidates for a given position."

The challenges of the first job accompany the professional, regardless of their area of training, during the first few months of their career. From then on, all the learning and support from the team they will be part of is of fundamental importance for this start. In this phase of initiation, the way in which the new graduate will face the challenges of the new profession can influence the development of their work. For newly qualified nurses, the feeling of insecurity in the face of difficulties is a challenge that runs through the admission process and continues during their adaptation to the health service (SOUZA et al., 2014).

Challenges can be seen as a highly stressful event, but they can also provide the possibility of transforming any difficult situation into growth and development. According to Souza et al. (2014), the transition from being a student to a professional can lead to a number of feelings, which can be described as a syndrome called "reality shock"; this occurs when the new graduate is unable to put into practice the knowledge gained during their degree.

In the field of nursing, it's important to note that working as a nurse, which is assigned by institutions to recent graduates, involves taking over an entire nursing team. This task can be extremely stressful and exhausting, even for a well-trained professional, as in many circumstances the nurse has to lead professionals who have worked for a long time. Therefore, the beginning of the nursing professional's activities can be marked by difficulties and prejudices in relation to lack of experience, young age, lack of leadership and technical skills and lack of support and structure from the employer (SOUZA et al., 2014).

Currently, nursing accounts for more than 50% of employment in the health sector. The Osvaldo Cruz Foundation (Fiocruz) and the Federal Nursing Council (COFEN) carried out a national survey on the profile of Brazilian nursing, in which 10.1% of the participants reported having experienced unemployment before the survey, which contradicts the consensus that the health sector, unlike other labor-intensive sectors, does not feel the effects of the crisis that is currently shaking the employability index (CASTAGNA, 2016).

It is therefore necessary to broaden our knowledge of nursing graduates in order to carry out and complement the evaluation of the teaching-learning process, with the aim of understanding the institution's training potential, the demands of society, the end product of the pedagogical work and the absorption of these professionals into the world of work (JESUS; GOMES; SPILERE, 2011).

Therefore, "[...] knowing the professional trajectory of graduates is a way of analyzing, understanding and reflecting on issues related to higher nursing education and the characteristics inherent in the job market" (COLENCI; BERTI, 2012, p. 159).

In this context, the general objective of this study is to characterize the profile and the difficulties encountered by nurses in the academic-professional transition, in order to verify whether the undergraduate education contemplates the needs of professional practice in the view of the graduates. The research is justified because collecting and reflecting on information about this profile could contribute to reflecting on the world of work of nurses today, helping to (re)direct their methodological resources, as well as providing input for proposals to improve the curriculum of the course under analysis.

2 OBJECTIVES

2.1 GENERAL OBJECTIVE

To characterize the profile and difficulties encountered by nurses in the academic-professional transition.

2.2 SPECIFIC OBJECTIVES

- To draw up a profile of the nurses who graduated from the university in this study in terms of gender, age and place of work.

- To check, from the point of view of the graduates, whether the degree program meets the needs of professional practice.

3 LITERATURE REVIEW

3.1 THE CHALLENGES OF THE WORLD OF WORK

Entering the world of work is a dream of young Brazilians, and having a successful career is part of their professional fulfillment. As a result of major political and technological changes, today's world of work is more demanding, requiring professional training in order to meet the standards required by companies (PAULA, 2012).

In today's globalized world and with growing technological advances in the health sector, the world of work demands new ways of constructing knowledge, requiring a new model for training professionals to be able to attend to the health of the population. This reality requires training institutions to improve their teaching in order to train professionals with competencies and skills (SILVA et al., 2010).

In this context, the relevance of the National Curricular Guidelines (DCN) for the Nursing Course to guide the profession in this new world of work is highlighted. The profile of the graduate should be that of a professional with a generalist, humanist, critical and reflective education, qualified to practice nursing, based on scientific and intellectual rigor and ethical principles. In addition to meeting social health needs, ensuring comprehensive care, quality and humanization of care, inserting themselves into the world of work (SILVA et al., 2010).

Thus, the challenge of the transition from academia to the work field is often a distressing process for recent graduates, and concern about this moment is something commonly observed in undergraduates and graduates; there is often obvious anxiety about having to take on the responsibilities attributed to the profession they have chosen, without the supervision they had when they were students (JESUS et al., 2013).

For educators, the great challenge is to train professionals who are able to respond to the demands of a complex society and enter a competitive world of work; thus, training should not only focus on entry and permanence in the world of work, but also emphasize a humanistic education that promotes the construction of critical, autonomous subjects with the capacity for transformation (JESUS et al., 2013).

As a result of the increase in the availability of new jobs in the nursing field over the last few decades, new higher education nursing schools have been opened, thus launching a significant number of graduates into the world of work. The consequences of this expansion have been a decrease in the average salary of the profession and professionals who are subject to low salaries and precarious conditions in order to maintain an employment relationship (NETO et al., 2014).

3.2 BRIEF HISTORY OF THE INSTITUTION AND THE DEGREE COURSE IN NURSING AT THE UNIVERSITY OF WESTERN SANTA CATARINA (UNOESC)

Unoesc defines itself as a multi-campus educational institution, which emerges from the technological and educational requirements of the region, with the aim of participating in the development of the West and Mid-West of Santa Catarina (UNIVERSIDADE DO OESTE DE SANTA CATARINA, 1991).

It emerged at the end of the 1960s, and its unification took place with three educational foundations existing in the region: Fundaçao Educacional do Oeste Catarinense (FUOC), Fundaçao Educacional e Empresarial do Alto do Vale do Rio do Peixe (Femarp) and Fundaçao de Ensino para o Desenvolvimento do Oeste (Fundeste). Later, Unoesc, Fundaçao Educacional do Extremo-Oeste de Santa Catarina (Funoesc) and Fundaçao Educacional dos Municipios do Alto Irani (FEMAI) were integrated (UNIVERSIDADE DO OESTE DE SANTA CATARINA, 2016).

Thus, it was authorized to implement its university project in 1991, "In 1996 we were recognized as a university by the State Education Council, and consequently accredited by the Ministry of Education" (UNIVERSIDADE DO OESTE DE SANTA CATARINA, 2016).

According to the University, the institution is currently:

> One of the largest institutions driving development, research and socio-cultural and educational perspectives in the regions it covers, its geographical area consists of approximately 118 municipalities and more than 1 million people, in a geographical area that runs from Santa Cecilia, in the central plateau of Santa Catarina to the border with Argentina, reaching the southwest of Paraná and the northwest of Rio Grande do Sul, made up of five campuses: Joaçaba, Videira, Xanxerê, Sao Miguel do Oeste and Chapecó; and the units: Capinzal, Campos Novos, Fraiburgo, Pinhalzinho, Maravilha and Sao José do Cedro(UNIVERSIDADE DO OESTE DE SANTA CATARINA, 2016, p.1).

The Nursing Degree Course at the Fundaçao Educacional dos Municipios do Alto Irani was recognized by the Ministry of Education (MEC) through Ministerial Order No. 253 of February 17, 1994, published in the Official Gazette of February 18, 1994, and renewed by Ministerial Order No. 436 of November 11, 2002, published in the Official Gazette of the State of Santa Catarina on November 12, 2002 (UNIVERSIDADE DO OESTE DE SANTA CATARINA, 2009).

The Nursing course began at Unoesc Joaçaba in 2006, linked to the former Area of Biological and Health Sciences, now the Area of Life Sciences. This course offers 40 places per year, full-time (afternoon and evening), with generalist training and a focus on public health (DALLACOSTA; MAKOWSKI; TOMASI, 2016); it lasts five years, spread over 10 semester phases, with practical classes during the day and theoretical/practical classes at night, totaling 4,005 hours (UNIVERSIDADE DO OESTE DE SANTA CATARINA, 2009).

According to the Nursing Course Pedagogical Project, the course's mission is to train nurses committed to the ethical, political and technical-scientific principles of the profession, capable of proposing and defending public policies and programs aimed at the population's healthy living process, with the defense and consolidation of nursing as a social practice as its guiding axis (UNIVERSIDADE DO OESTE DE SANTA CATARINA, 2009).

The course met the need to train nurses due to the shortage of these professionals in the city and region. The first class of nurses from Unoesc in Joaçaba graduated at the end of 2009, and there are currently six classes of graduates, totaling 192 nurses over the course's 10 years (DALLACOSTA; MAKOWSKI; TOMASI, 2016).

Unoesc seeks to encourage its graduates to find opportunities in the world of work to change the reality of the profession, changing the scenario of institutions in the region, which, until some time ago, were coordinated by mid-level professionals and the profession was practiced empirically. This scenario has undergone several changes since these graduates entered the world of work, since institutions now have professionals trained to provide quality care at different levels of assistance (DALLACOSTA; MAKOWSKI; TOMASI, 2016).

3.3 HISTORY OF NURSING AND THE IMPORTANCE OF KNOWING THE PROFILE OF GRADUATES

The historical foundations guide and underpin the current scenario. In order to understand the reality of nursing education in Brazil, it is important to review its trajectory, trends and contradictions. Based on the assumption that the quality of the nursing professional and, consequently, their insertion in the world of work is largely linked to appropriate professional preparation, it is necessary to know how this trajectory was to qualify nurses (COLENCI, 2009).

The nursing profession emerged from the evolution of health practices throughout history. The first health practices were instinctive, which, at the first moment of civilization, guaranteed the maintenance of human survival; they were more directed at women's work, but over time having mastery of the means of healing meant power, so man combined this knowledge with mysticism, taking possession of it (OGUISSO, 2014).

As for nursing, historical references are related to the practice of home births and the simple work of women who shared activities in temples with priests (OGUISSO, 2014).

However, over the years, nursing stopped being based so much on common sense and mysticism and began to consider health practices from the point of view of the political and economic system of capitalist society. Nursing therefore emerged as an institutionalized professional activity, beginning with the Industrial Revolution of the 16th century, culminating in the emergence of modern nursing in the 19th century in England (JESUS et al., 2010).

In Florence, Italy, in 1820, Florence Nightgale was born, the daughter of a British high society family, who became the pioneer of modern nursing, gaining greater visibility with her participation as a volunteer in the Crimean War in 1854, in which she implemented improvements in the wards of the Hospital in Scutari, contributing to the rescue of sanitary conditions in relation to the environment and hygiene (LOPES; SANTOS, 2010).

Florence raised the *status of* this profession through the qualification of care through her theoretical and universal teachings, which were based on the empowerment of her subjectivity, becoming a theoretician and a reference for the integrality of health work (OGUISSO, 2014).

Also in 1860, in Victorian England, the nursing team was categorized into *Nurses* and *Lady-Nurses*, which led to fragmented care, since the *ladies were* responsible for teaching and supervision, and the *nurses for* manual tasks; they lived and worked in the hospital throughout the course, received a salary and, after the course, were assigned to direct patient care (SOUZA et al., 2006).

In Brazil, professionalization began in 1890, with the founding of the Professional School for Nurses at the Hospital dos Alienados, and with the emergence of psychiatry in the country, currently the Alfredo Pinto School in Rio de Janeiro (OGUISSO, 2014).

Among the pioneers who marked the history of nursing in Brazil, Ana Justina Ferreira Nery stood out as a pioneer of the profession after taking part in the Paraguayan War as a volunteer, caring for wounded soldiers alongside her two sons and two brothers; She received two notable honors: the first, as the mother of Brazilians, she was received by Emperor Dom Pedro II when she returned from the war, bringing with her three orphans of dead soldiers whom she raised as her own children, and the second when the National School of Public Health was renamed the Ana Nery Nurses School (OGUISSO, 2014).

On August 5, 1949, Law No. 775/49 was passed, which standardized nursing education in Brazil with a duration of 36 months, and in the same year, Decree No. 27.426/49, which directed the curriculum for the training of nurses (SANTOS, 2003).

Since then, curricular changes in nursing education have become necessary in order to achieve practice with proposals that are close to reality and in order to make students aware that professional training is a process of permanent construction (DIAS; GUARIENTE; BELEI, 2004).

According to Rodrigues, Conterno and Guedes (2015, p. 29), "[...] academic training alone is not enough to guarantee insertion into the world of work and qualified professional performance, however, when of high quality, it can be a positive element."

This highlights the importance of knowing the professional trajectory of graduates, as a way of analyzing, understanding and reflecting on issues relating to higher nursing education and the characteristics inherent in the job market (COLENCI; BERTI, 2012).

Considering that today's world of work has growing demands for productivity and quality, is flexible and unstable, making the implementation of training and workforce management models based on professional competencies increasingly widespread (DELUIZ, 2001), the university where this study was carried out states that the graduate profile should be:

> A generalist, humanist, critical and reflective professional, qualified to exercise the profession, based on scientific and intellectual rigor and based on ethical principles, acting on health problems and situations, qualified to develop health promotion actions in the management of health services and able to act with a sense of social responsibility and commitment to citizenship, as a promoter of the integral health of the human being and to act in the various areas of the labor market. (UNIVERSIDADE DO OESTE DE SANTA CATARINA, 2009, p. 11).

Since graduates represent the end product of universities, monitoring them contributes to the constant adaptation and transformation related to the world of work; for national health and education policy, they are the bridge between academia and the world of work, and their resourcefulness in it is one of the most important parameters of the quality of teaching (CARRIJO et al., 2007).

4 METHODOLOGY

A descriptive and exploratory study with a quantitative and qualitative approach, carried out with nursing graduates from a private higher education institution in the Midwest of Santa Catarina who completed their degree between 2009/2 and 2015/2, 2009 being the year in which the first class of the Nursing Course graduated.

Data was collected by means of a semi-structured questionnaire specially designed for this investigation (APPENDIX A), attached and sent via *e-mail* to the graduates, which were made available by the Nursing Course Coordination; in addition, the contacts also contained telephone numbers. In order to increase the sample of participants answering the questionnaire, we searched for all the graduates via social networks such as Facebook and WhatsApp, sending them an individual message inviting them to take part in the survey. Inclusion criteria were all academics who received contact via *e-mail* or social networks. Excluded from the study were students who had submitted their Course Conclusion Work (TCC) but had not yet completed their degree.

Open and closed questions were used to characterize the social and professional variables of the population investigated and to identify the difficulties in entering the world of work, as well as perceptions of training. The data was collected between June and July 2016 and stored on the Google Docs platform, which was automatically fed with the answers sent by each participant. The quantitative part was analyzed by absolute frequency and percentage, and the qualitative part by transcribing the experience reports.

This study complies with Resolution 466/12 and was submitted to the Ethics and Research Committee (CEP) of the Universidade do Oeste de Santa Catarina de Joaçaba, for approval under opinion no. 1.482.384 (APPENDIX A).

Graduates agreed to take part in the study by signing the Free and Informed Consent Form (FICF) (ANNEX B), which was returned to them either in person or as an electronic copy. In this way, participants were guaranteed anonymity and confidentiality of information. Anonymity was maintained by identifying them by the letter E (Egress), followed by a numerical order from 1 to 74.

5 RESULTS AND DISCUSSION

5.1 CHARACTERIZATION OF GRADUATES

Of the 194 graduates between 2009 and 2015, 190 were contacted, but only 74 (38.9%) responded to the questionnaire made available via *e-mail*.

Initially, the profile of the graduates was drawn up in terms of gender and age, as shown in Table 1.

Table 1 - Characterization of graduates according to gender and age group

Age	N	Female	%	Male	%
20 - 25	18	18	24,3	0	0,0
26 - 30	38	35	47,3	3	4,0
31 - 40	13	12	16,2	1	1,4
41 - 49	5	4	5,4	1	1,4
Total	74	69	93,2	5	6,8

Source: the author.

The majority were female, ranging in age from 20 to 49, with the 26 to 30 age group predominating in both sexes.

Corroborating this data, Oliveira, Tashima and Costa (2015), in a study carried out with the aim of finding out the perception of nursing graduates from a university in southern Brazil about the process of training for professional practice, showed similar data, in which 90% of the interviewees were women and the average age of the interviewees was 24.7±0.26 years.

Also, Cambiriba, Ferronato and Fontes (2014), in a private higher education institution in Paranà, with similar objectives to this study, found similar data, i.e. 77.3% of the participants were female, predominantly in the 22-30 age group.

Martins et al. (2006) state that one of the characteristics of nursing is that it is mostly practiced by women, and that it can be considered a feminine trait to carry out the work of caring. However, the demand from men for the profession has increased considerably over the years.

The predominance of women in nursing is justifiable, since historically the profession was practiced by religious orders in which the majority of health care activities were carried out by women in a charitable manner. Another factor that should be considered is the influence of Florence Nightingale in institutionalizing nursing as a profession for women, for which they are naturally prepared (LOPES; LEAL, 2005). For Lima, Vieira and Costa (2014), because the history of the profession is made up of women, this fact can make it difficult for male students to enter the profession, both by society and by the female majority that make up the category.

The Osvaldo Cruz Foundation (Fiocruz), in partnership with the Federal Nursing Council (COFEN), evaluated the profile of nursing in Brazil at national level in 2015. The data showed that the nursing team is predominantly female, comprising 84.6% women, and highlighted that even though it is a female category, there are 15% men, and it can be said that in nursing there is a trend towards masculinization of the category, with the growing increase of the male contingent in the composition (FUNDAÇÂO OSVALDO CRUZ, 2015).

Table 2 shows the municipality of residence and the municipality where these graduates work in the professional world.

Table 2 - Characterization of graduates according to municipality of residence and municipality of professional activity

Municipality	Residence	%	Work	%
Joaçaba	22	29.8	36	48.6
Herval d'Oeste	13	17.6	06	8.1
Campos Novos	03	4,0	02	2.7
Others	36	48.6	30	40.6

Source: the author.

It was found that many graduates remained in the municipality where they studied, and the majority work in Joaçaba. Of the 74 graduates, most live and/or work in municipalities close to Joaçaba, such as Luzerna and Caçador, as well as on the coast, in the state of Rio Grande do Sul and cities in Paranà.

The city of Joaçaba is located in the Midwest of Santa Catarina, which has approximately 370,000 inhabitants; according to IBGE data (2016), the city currently has 29,310 inhabitants, but is part of a micro-region with two other neighboring cities, Herval d'Oeste and Luzerna, which together have 28,027 inhabitants.

According to the Regional Nursing Council (COREN) (2016), 12,117 nurses were registered in the state of Santa Catarina in 2015; data from 2016 showed 12,586 registered nurses, of which 94 are nurses who live in the municipality of Joaçaba and 155 positions are held by nurses in this municipality.

Perhaps the reason for staying in the city is the jobs on offer and the quality of life it offers. There are two medium-sized hospitals in Joaçaba, as well as jobs in primary care, private clinics, institutes and secretariats linked to the state and federal governments. The Santa Terezinha University Hospital had its physical structure expanded, and this year saw the inauguration of the new building, which was named Torre Joao Paulo II, with 87 new beds, generating an increase in the workforce (RADIO CATARINENSE, 2016). According to Cancian (2016), the nursing coordinator at the Santa Terezinha University Hospital, the hospital currently employs 64 nurses (APPENDIX C).

Another relevant fact, according to Dallacosta, Makowski and Tomasi (2016), is that since the first graduating class, graduates have found job opportunities in the city and region, which has contributed to changing the reality of the profession, since these professionals have been implementing improvements in institutes, thus helping to provide quality care at the different levels of health care.

Table 3 shows the characterization of the graduates in terms of the year they completed their degree and their satisfaction with the learning they received during the course.

Table 3 - Characterization of graduates in terms of year of completion and satisfaction with their degree

				Satisfaction with the degree			
Year completed	Number of graduates	Number of graduates taking part	%	Full	Partial	Not very satisfied	Dissatisfied
2009/2	26	6	19,3	1	4	0	0
2010/2	31	6	19,3	2	4	0	0
2011/2	31	12	38,7	0	12	0	0
2013/1	46	23	50,0	7	15	1	0
2014/2	30	12	40,0	3	9	0	0
2015/2	26	15	57,7	3	13	0	0

Source: the author.

To date, Unoesc Joaçaba has graduated six classes in the Nursing undergraduate course; this survey included the participation of graduates from all the years in which graduation took place. The highest percentage of graduates taking part was from the 2015/2 graduating class. It should be noted that there was no graduation ceremony in 2012 due to a change in the curriculum matrix, which extended the student's training time.

When asked about their satisfaction with the learning they received during their degree, the partially satisfied index predominated in all years, while the highest number of fully satisfied graduates were from the class of 2013; there was also one graduate who was not very satisfied with the learning.

Graduates' satisfaction may be being met as a result of the training model, which is meeting what is expected in the context of professional practice and the world of work. Therefore, graduate satisfaction is a factor that should be explored and becomes an indicator of the quality of both their training and service provision, putting into practice what they have learned best in their training (MEIRA; KURCGANT, 2009).

Graph 1 - Commitment to learning during the course

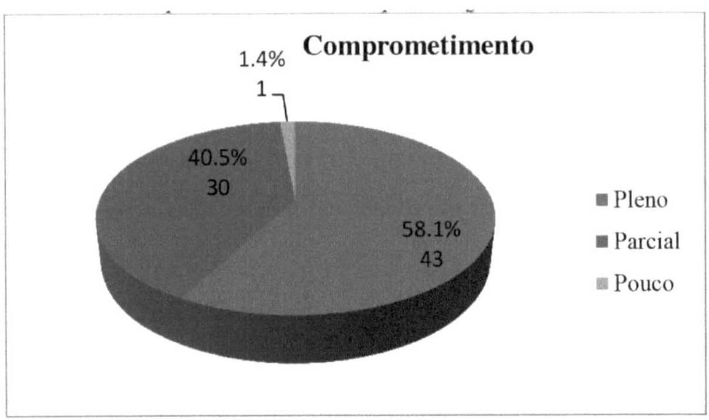

Source: the author.

When asked about their commitment to learning during their degree, the answers showed high levels of full commitment, followed by partial commitment. However, one graduate said he had little commitment to learning, perhaps due to professional frustration or a wrong choice of course.

Moreira et al. (2016), in a descriptive study on the difficulties and challenges faced by nurses when they were admitted to hospital units, showed that the highest percentage of interviewees reported that the academic qualification was productive for their insertion into the world of work, demonstrating that dedication to learning facilitates insertion into the world of work. Mattosinho et al. (2010) emphasize that these professionals, regardless of difficult and adverse situations, manage to cope and carry out their activities in the best possible way and with good judgment.

We also identified the occupations that the graduates held before studying nursing, as shown in Table 4.

Table 4 - Occupation of graduates before graduation

Occupation before graduation	Frequency	%
Nursing Technician	25	33,8
Student	18	24,3
Trainee	08	10,8
Administrative Assistant	08	10,8
Others	15	20,3

Source: the author.

In relation to their professional occupation before graduating, it can be seen that the majority worked in the area as technical professionals, others only studied and among those who ticked the other option, they listed the following areas in the highest proportion: receptionist, teacher, sales assistant, community health worker and farmer.

Similar data were found in studies carried out by Colenci and Berti (2012) and Moreira et al. (2016) with graduates of a Nursing Degree Course at a private institution, in which 17.30% and 50%, respectively, worked as nursing technicians before graduating.

Machado et al. (2016a) analyzed the general aspects of the professional training of nursing staff in Brazil who have active registration with the Federal Nursing Council and highlighted that 1/3 (31.4%) of the nursing contingent took a technical or auxiliary nursing course before graduating, and that 78.1% showed interest in continuing their studies by graduating in nursing, which confirms the value that education has been receiving as a decisive factor in improving insertion in the job market.

Maier and Mattos (2016) report that the activities of students at university concomitant with those inherent to working in the health area is a reality, as nursing technicians have more often than not sought a degree in the same area, needing the salary to support themselves and/or their families, requiring willpower not to give up, as staying in school is conditional on working, and the reason that leads students to follow this path is to improve their financial conditions.

According to Medina and Takahashi (2003), in their study 38.3% of the graduates worked as nursing technicians before graduating, and one of the results was that previous experience in nursing facilitated learning, both theoretically and practically.

Table 5 - Characteristics of graduates in terms of professional activity

	Variable	Frequency	%
Works in the field	Yes	67	90,5
	No	07	9,5
	1	42	56,8
How many jobs do you have	2	23	31,1
	+2	02	2,7
	Does not work	07	9,4
	Morning	09	12,2
Work shift	Afternoon	04	5,4
	Evening	09	12,2
	Two shifts	52	70,2

Source: the author.

Although the majority are working in the field and have only one job, what is striking is the length of time they work. The data shows a high number of professionals who work two or more shifts.

Corroborating this, Silva (2016), in an analysis of the results of the survey Profile of nursing in Brazil, with the aim of suggesting improvements in the category, found similar data, since 58% of nurses reported having only one job, and 32.6% declared having two or three activities. The author also points out that work overload has led to illness and the need for treatment.

Oliveira et al. (2014), in their study, analyzed the professional insertion of 45 nursing graduates from a state public university in Ceará and found that 44.4% of nurses work more than 40 hours, usually with more than one job.

Due to low salaries and unfavorable economic situations, nursing workers often need to work several jobs, taking on double shifts, which harms their quality of life (LIMA et al., 2016). In a study by Ferreira (2015), this is also confirmed, since among the stressors for nurses is the double working day, which causes damage to health and illness.

Currently, the category has no salary floor, and Bill 459/2015 has been in progress since 2015, which establishes a salary floor for nurses, nursing technicians, nursing assistants and midwives. The bill's authors argue that health professionals work more than one job in order to earn a decent wage, but that this is often not achieved, and that the stressful working day irreparably compromises both the health of the professional and the quality of patient care. Approval of this bill will bring better working conditions for professionals who, by receiving remuneration commensurate with their responsibilities, will be able to practice their trade in just one establishment, as well as having their professional value enhanced (CÂMARA DOS DEPUTADOS, 2015).

Table 6 - Categorization of graduates in terms ofimprovement courses already completed

Refresher course	Frequency	%
Specialization	59	79.7
Master's Degree	04	5.4
No courses	10	13.5
Other	01	1.4

Source: the author.

After graduating, the search for further training was observed, and the most common option was specialization, followed by no courses.

Corroborating the data, Oliveira et al. (2016) investigated the professional trajectory of nursing graduates from a private university center in Teresina, Piaui, and almost all the interviewees who said they had taken another course after completing their undergraduate degree in nursing, 80.4%

(n=160), took a specialization course, 4% (n=8) took a master's degree and 14% (n=28) ticked the other option, which refers to another undergraduate course.

Similar data was also found in a study carried out by Püschel, Inacio and Pucci (2009) at the Nursing School of the Federal University of Sao Paulo (USP), in which they characterized the graduates of the Nursing Degree Course, from 2000 to 2005, and found that 63.4% of the graduates had taken some kind of specialization course.

The National Education Guidelines and Bases Law (LDB), Law No. 9.394/1996, assigns two levels of education to national education, Basic Education and Higher Education, which is broken down into undergraduate and postgraduate. With regard to postgraduate studies, the LDB, in article 44, defines:

> Art. 44 Higher education will include the following courses and programs: [...]
>
> III - postgraduate courses, comprising master's and doctoral programs, specialization courses, further training and others, open to candidates who have graduated from undergraduate courses and meet the requirements of the educational institutions (BRASIL, 2016).

In a study, Silva (2016) points out that the Federal Nursing Council (COFEN) presented a basic document entitled *Public Policy Proposals for Nursing,* based on data from the Profile of Nursing in Brazil survey, and highlighted the existence of a high number of professionals in the category with specialization.

It is believed that most of the graduates surveyed sought professional qualification in order to stand out in the competitive world of work, specializing in their area of activity, or to train for future positions for which they have greater affinity, interest and dedication, with the aim of professional fulfillment.

For Vall, Pereira and Friesen (2009, p. 8), "[...] taking a specialization course is an important fact, since having nurses who are specialists in different areas of activity only increases the prestige and respect for the profession in the job market."

Table 7 shows the areas in which the nurses are working and their level of professional satisfaction.

Table 7 - Field of work and professional satisfaction

Job satisfaction										
			Very satisfied				SatisfiedUnsatisfied			Very
Graduates			unsatisfied							
	n	%	n	%	n	%	n	%	n	%
Hospital	36	48.6	13	36.1	22	61,1	01	2.8	00	0.0
ESF	14	18.9	03	21.4	09	64.3	02	14.3	00	0.0

Teaching	07	9.5	03	42.9	04	57.1	00	0.0	00	0.0
SAMU	01	1.3	00	0.0	01	100	00	0.0	00	0.0
Clinic	04	5.4	01	25.0	03	75.0	00	0.0	00	0.0
Other	09	12.2	05	55.6	04	44.4	00	0.0	00	0.0
Does not work	03	4.1	00	0.0	00	0,0	00	0.0	03	100

Source: the author.

Notes: n: Number of graduates;

ESF : Family Health Strategy;

SAMU: Mobile Emergency Care Service.

According to Souza et al. (2014), the choice of profession is an individual's own choice and requires knowledge of the aspects inherent in the career and the function to be performed in professional life, as well as new opportunities with the emergence of new jobs.

The data in Table 7 shows that the majority of nurses work in hospitals and say they are satisfied or very satisfied with their current situation, followed by those who work in the Family Health Strategy, the majority of whom say they are very satisfied, showing that, in general, nurses are personally satisfied with their professional work. The minority of professionals were dissatisfied.

Similar data was found by Oliveira (2016) in a study that investigated the career path of nursing graduates from a private higher education institution in the city of Teresina, in which 64.21% of graduates are working in the hospital area, 6.84% work in basic health units, 21.05% are linked to teaching and/or research, and 3.16% work in science.

In another study, Maia (2014) researched the profile of nursing graduates from a Federal University in Piaui and found similar data; employment in the hospital sector was the most frequent, with 46.4%, followed by the public health sector with 23.5%.

Pava and Neves (2011) say that since the emergence of the first nursing schools, there has been a need to train nurses to treat the sick in hospital environments. Corroborating these results, Colenci and Berti (2012) state that new jobs have emerged as a result of the implementation of the Unified Health System (SUS) in the country, such as the Family Health Strategy, which has become one of the best options today.

The data is justified by the fact that the hospital world requires a greater number of professionals, since a hospital unit needs at least four nurses, because they work continuous shifts (depending on the level of care provided, this number is greater), while an ESF team only needs one nurse to work, so it is expected that the insertion will occur more in the hospital area (CONSELHO FEDERAL DE

ENFERMAGEM, 2004).

With regard to the level of job satisfaction, most of the participants in the survey reported being satisfied. According to Nunes et al. (2010, p. 255), job satisfaction is:

> The sum of the different elements that make up the personal and professional world, as well as the result of the worker's assessment of their work, a set of elements that contribute to satisfaction, such as: recognition, happiness, respect, the work environment and working conditions, being necessary to enjoy what you do, have adequate remuneration, a good relationship with the team, the possibility of growth and professional recognition.

This would therefore justify the percentage of dissatisfaction, which is related to not working as a nurse and perhaps not being professionally fulfilled.

Morais et al. (2014), with the aim of identifying the factors that generate job dissatisfaction among nurses at a university hospital in the interior of the state of Paranà, through the participants' testimonies, revealed that overload generates job dissatisfaction.

Furthermore, Malagutti (2012, p. 70) states:

> Since the time of our forerunner Florence, nursing has been evolving and conquering different areas of activity every day, becoming increasingly diversified and comprehensive in different areas of professional activity. The advance of technology, coupled with globalization, means that nurses in the modern era are increasingly focused on know-how, focusing their skills on quality nursing care in the current health scenario, be it care, administrative, educational and/or managerial.

When they left school, the graduates of the research institution followed different paths to find a job; the aim of this qualitative study was to analyze the opinions of the graduates in relation to the difficulties they faced in finding their first job, criticisms of their academic training and what could be improved during their studies that would contribute to their professional performance.

According to the reports below, the majority had no difficulty in getting their first job, especially those already working in the area as nursing technicians, who were absorbed by the institutions as nurses. They entered the profession by various means, and there were cases in which their first job came about as a result of taking part in a public examination while they were studying for their degree. When asked about the difficulties, they reported:

None, because I was already absorbed by the institution where I already worked as a nursing technician. (E20, E68)

No difficulties, several opportunities came up, I chose the most suitable one. (E24, E30)

I didn't have any difficulties, because I passed a public examination. (E67)

Very little difficulty, I took three exams and passed all three. (E56)

When I graduated I soon got my first job as a nurse because I took a public exam and two months after graduating I was already working in the field. (E44)

The fact that most of the graduates reported that they had no difficulty in entering the world of work, and that most of them were already working as nursing technicians, means that the technical level is a facilitator for entering the world of work and helped them to be absorbed by the institutions in which they worked. This fact, according to Souza et al. (2014), becomes a positive factor in the face of the difficulties experienced, since they knew the techniques, routines and professionals who worked there, reducing the stress of the new job, the fear of the unknown and insecurity, facilitating professional integration.

The lack of professional experience was a difficulty, as it is currently a factor required by institutions when hiring professionals.

Lack of experience in nursing, although I didn't find it very difficult. (E66)

No experience (E5, 6, 7, 9, 13)

Machado et al. (2016b) carried out a study with nursing professionals in Brazil who are registered with the nursing council, analyzing the general aspects of the job market for nursing staff in terms of the way in which they are inserted into the various health sectors and highlighted that, among nurses, 21% related the lack of professional experience as a difficulty in getting their first job.

Among the reasons for dissatisfaction are the low salaries offered by institutions in our region, since nursing does not have a salary floor, which is why some graduates do not work in the area and declare themselves professionally dissatisfied.

I'm still without a job. The offers are totally unsatisfactory. Spending a fortune on your degree only to arrive on the job market and find yourself in a totally undervalued class, where salaries are shameful [...]. (E8)

Low pay, very low. (E15)

I'm not working as a nurse at the moment because my salary is very low, but I'm interested in taking part in public tenders in the future. (E36)

As a result of the category not having a salary floor, Silva (2016) says that Brazilian nurses are subjected to precarious and unacceptable salaries, being the least paid category in the health area, stressing the importance of approving Bill 459/2015, referring to the salary floor.

In addition, the categorization of the professional class by the institutions was also cited as a hindrance to entering the profession. Since it was recognized as a profession, nursing has had hierarchical divisions. Currently, nurses, nursing technicians and nursing assistants are recognized, **of which there** are no subdivisions.

Being a new graduate is complicated everywhere, and today with these trainee programs we are forced to accept. It was difficult for me to accept, because I've always maintained that I don't agree with junior nurses [...] (E55).

The existence of the "Junior Nurse" function, because it devalues undergraduates. (E28)

Law n. 7.498, of 1986, which regulates the practice of nursing, states that:

Art. 2 Nursing and its ancillary activities may only be practiced by legally qualified persons registered with the Regional Nursing Council with jurisdiction in the area where the practice takes place.

Sole Paragraph. Nursing is carried out exclusively by nurses, nursing technicians, nursing assistants and midwives, subject to their respective qualifications.

When asked, the majority said they had no criticisms of their training. Among the other graduates, the majority report that the course is geared towards a hospital emphasis, hindering other possibilities for nurses to work in public health, despite the fact that the PPC has collective health as its conceptual axis Some procedures, technical and managerial skills are also pointed out as insufficient, since theoretical teaching takes up a large part of the workload.

Graduation geared towards a hospital-centered view. (E4)

During the course, I realized that some subjects had few practical lessons. As a result, when I graduated I found it difficult to deal with some situations. (E39)

There could be more practical lessons. (E13, 22, 27, 70,71)

There was a lack of management in the ESF internships, which focused too much on prevention and techniques [...] forgetting the bureaucratic responsibilities of nurses. (E5)

Meira and Kurcgant (2009), in a study that aimed to relate the importance attributed to undergraduate teaching with the assumptions of the National Curriculum Guidelines (DCNs) for nursing, suggest strengthening interdisciplinary practice and point to the need to improve the distribution of content and workload of subjects aimed at training administrative skills.

According to Rodrigues, Conterno and Guedes (2015), the student's training is procedural and will take place throughout their professional career. It is therefore the student's responsibility to take on the role of subject of their own education, given the differentiated and rich spaces of knowledge in which they will have to participate.

Practical classes in laboratories have been offered since the early stages of the course at this institution, with the subjects of Nursing Practice I, II and III in its curriculum, totaling 240 hours, which allows theoretical knowledge to be correlated with practice, for which the Skills Laboratory is available, located on campus II of the university, where students have equipment and mannequins suitable for training different skills and nursing procedures during classes and remains available to students whenever necessary (UNIVERSIDADE DO OESTE DE SANTA CATARINA, 2009).

In subjects such as Women's Health, Adult Health and Children's Health, students also correlate theoretical learning with laboratory practice, and in the Supervised Internship I, II and III component, especially in phase 10ª , students must carry out management activities, such as action plans and interventions in the internship sector, as provided for in the teaching plans (UNIVERSIDADE DO OESTE DE SANTA CATARINA, 2009).

It is known that some concepts are only exposed, either because it is difficult to have access to the experience or because of the lack of time in training. Another aspect observed in the questions is the teacher's responsibility, pointing to a lack of knowledge and professional experience.

I believe that in order to work in teaching, we need to be prepared, and some teachers have left something to be desired.

Teachers with higher qualifications in the area of teaching, experience, technical and scientific knowledge for the subject they work on. (E29)

Some teachers with little experience, especially during internships. (E68)

Some teachers have no knowledge of the area. (E48)

Lack of teachers who have worked in hospitals before teaching. (E6)

Based on the above reports, the graduates' view is that teachers are unprepared. According to Backes, Moyà and Prado (2011), the unpreparedness of teachers influences the professional training process, and continuing training is necessary.

For Junges and Behrens (2015, p. 286), "[...] Pedagogical training allows university professors to look at their pedagogical practice, interpret it and recreate it, making it a source of learning from a perspective of change and innovation."

When asked what could be improved during their undergraduate studies to help them work in the world of work, the interviewees listed the following: more practical classes, qualified teachers, especially in the field of internships, greater demands from teachers on students, dedication on the part of students and more incentives for research.

Firstly, the interest of the students, I think people think that everything in nursing is easy and they don't dedicate themselves as they should. [...] there's a lack of commitment, students should be charged a lot more. We're working with lives and today I see that to be a nurse you have to be 100% dedicated. If there was a greater demand, I'm sure that professionals would be better prepared, more mature and with a higher level of knowledge. (E23)

Invest in teaching, more qualified teachers. (E68)

Encouraging research (E36)

Encourage scientific research, nursing as a science, not just care. (E58)

[...] research groups with the University Hospital. (E11)

Reports on the lack of incentives for research were mentioned by three graduates in 2009 and 2011; in subsequent years the subject was not mentioned, perhaps because the undergraduate program is encouraging its students to do research.

and the availability of scientific initiation programs offered by educational institutions and the government.

According to Pereira (2014), it is in the classroom that questions arise and where the teacher must awaken in the students attitudes of search and investigation, through the exchange of knowledge, because in order to have research it is necessary to have questions. Araùjo et al. (2015, p. 9181) point out that "[...] research contributes to academic development and professional training, providing the maturing of ideas and broadening the critical vision of these students", but there are still few higher education institutes that have specific programs to encourage research, especially in private colleges.

In view of the above, Dallacosta, Makowski and Tomasi (2016) point out that the Pedagogical Project of the Nursing Course includes the importance of articulating the three basic pillars of academic training: teaching, research and extension. With a view to fostering teaching and learning among students, the professors of the Unoesc faculty created the Nursing Studies and Research Group (GEPE) in 2015, which is recent and encourages students and professors to become researchers.

In the following statement, one of the graduates from the first cohort says that when she took her degree, there was a need for changes to meet the needs of the working world, which she has noticed over the years. She also says that professional development and success depend on one's objectives.

As it was at the beginning of the course, some changes needed to be made, which I realize have been made today!" (E23)

The search for improvement in the profession is a whole context that depends a lot on each professional, their commitment, dedication, study. Health professionals will always have something to add to their profession, it depends on their objectives!(E32)

The Undergraduate Nursing Course at Unoesc Joaçaba has completed 10 years and is constantly improving. It is clear that one of the objectives of the teaching staff is to train professionals who are able to face the world of work with knowledge, skills and attitude, based on the ethical principles of the profession; the graduates have a mission to make nursing recognized and to carry out the profession based on scientific knowledge, providing quality assistance and humanized care. Therefore, in order to have a successful career, you first need to study, work hard, be focused and, above all, be passionate about what you do.

6 FINAL CONSIDERATIONS

The results show that the profile of the graduates is that of young adults, with a predominance of females aged between 26 and 30. Many of the graduates remained in the municipality where they studied, and the majority work in Joaçaba. Of the 74 graduates who took part, most live and/or work in municipalities close to Joaçaba, such as Luzerna and Caçador, and on the coast, in the state of Rio Grande do Sul and in cities in Paranâ.

The graduates are satisfied with the learning they received during their degree and reported full and partial commitment to learning during the course.

Most of them worked in the nursing field as technicians before graduating. Currently, 90.5% of the graduates who took part in the survey work as nurses, the majority have only one job and a large number of them work two shifts, mostly in hospitals, and they say they are satisfied and/or very satisfied professionally.

After graduating, many people undertook professional training, of which 79.7% did a specialization course, 5.4% did a master's degree, and one respondent ticked the other box.

Most of them had no trouble getting their first job, but many cited lack of professional experience, low salaries and the categorization of professional class by institutions as obstacles. They entered the world of work in different ways, such as through public examinations during their undergraduate studies, and many were absorbed by the institution where they worked, especially those who worked as nursing technicians.

Their criticisms of the undergraduate program were the hospital-centric approach, the low number of hours of practical classes and the lack of experience of the teachers, especially in internships.

They pointed to some factors that could contribute even more to their integration into the world of work, such as an increase in practical classes, qualified teachers, especially in the internship fields, greater pressure from teachers on their students, as well as commitment and dedication on the part of the students.

It was concluded that the majority of graduates are in the world of work and are professionally fulfilled; the course offers the conditions to compete professionally, but attention must be paid to market needs and trends.

It is hoped that this study will broaden reflections on how to face these challenges of the academic-professional transition in nursing and that new teaching and practice strategies will be devised. It is suggested that, for internship fields, teachers with knowledge and experience in the area, an increase in the number of hours of practical classes within the possibilities allowed by the curriculum, more pressure from teachers on their students, and, it should be emphasized, knowledge is acquired when both sides are committed.

REFERENCES

ARAÙJO, Alyne Màgda de Lima et al. Pesquisa cientifica na graduaçao em enfermagem e sua importamento na formaçao profissional. **Revista enfermagem UFPE on-line** , Recife, v. 9, n. 9, p. 9180-9187, set. 2015. Available at: < http://www.revista.ufpe.br/revistaenfermagem/index.php/revista/article/download/8106/130 25 >. Access em: 13 out. 2016.

BACKES, Vania Marli Schubert; MOYA, Jose Luis Medina; PRADO, Marta Lenise do Processo de construçao do construção do construção do construção pedagògico do docente universitàrio de enfermagem. **Revista Latino Americana de Enfermagem** , v. 19, n. 2, Mar./Apr. 2011. Available at: <http://r.search.yahoo.com/_ylt=A0LEVj1Wnv5XIGwAKP0f7At.;_ylu=X3oDMTByMG04Z 2o2BHNlYwNzcgRwb3MDMQRjb2xvA2JmMQR2dGlkAw-- /RV=2/RE=1476333270/RO=10/RU=http%3 a%2f% 2fwww.scielo.br%2fpdf%2frlae%2fv19n 2%2fpt_26.pdf/RK=0/RS=ghJwwhEx7ECX0kMKoHDjbBWdXjU->. Access em: 12 out. 2016.

BRAZIL. Lei n. 7,498, of July 25 , 1986. Dispoe sobre a regulamentaçao do exercicio da enfermagem, e dà outras providências. **Diàrio Oficial da União** , Brasilia, DF, June 25 , 1986. Available at: < http://www.planalto.gov.br/ccivil_03/Leis/L7498.htm >. Access em: 12 out. 2016.

BRAZIL. Lei n. 9,394, of 20 de dezembro de 1996. Estabelece as Diretrizes e Bases da Educaçao. **Diàrio Oficial da União** , Brasilia, DF, 21 Dec. 2016. Available at: < https://www.planalto.gov.br/ccivil_03/Leis/L9394.htm >. Access em: 07 out. 2016.

CHAMBER DOS DEPUTADOS. **Projeto de Lei n. 459/2015** . Dispoe sobre a Piso Salarial do Enfermeiro, do Tècnico de Enfermagem, do Auxiliar de Enfermagem e da Parteira. Brasilia, DF, 25 Feb. 2015. Available at: < http://www.camara.gov.br/proposicoesWeb/fichadetramitacao?idProposicao=949035 >. Access em: 15 out. 2016.

CAMBIRIBA, Thayse Fernanda Colombo; FERRONATO, Aline Ferreira; FONTES, Katya Biagio. Percepçoes de egressos de enfermagem frente a inserçao no mercado de trabalho. **Arquivo de Ciência da Saùde UNIPAR** , Umuarama, v. 18, n. 1, p. 27-32, Jan./Apr. 2014. Available at: < http://revistas.unipar.br/index.php/saude/article/view/5155/2981 >. Access em: 08 out. 2016.

CANCIAN, Leandra. **Enfermeiros atuantes no Hospital Universitario Santa Terezinha** [Mensagem pessoal]. Message received by < renata.dalberto@hotmail.com > em 04 out. 2016

CASTAGNA, Valdirlei. Mercado de trabalho da enfermagem: general aspects. **Enfermagem em Foco** , v. 7, p. 35-62, 2016. Ediçao Especial. Available at: <

http://revista.portalcofen.gov.br/index.php/enfermagem/article/view/694/304 >. Access em: 15 out. 2016.

CARRIJO, Clarissa Irineu de Sousa. et al. A empregabilidade de egressos de um curso de graduaçao em enfermagem. **Revista de Enfermagem UERJ** , Rio de Janeiro, v. 15, n. 3, p. 356-363, July/September. 2007. Available at: < http://www.facenf.uerj.br/v15n3/v15n3a06.pdf >. Accessed: 21 Jun 2016.

COLLENCI, Raquel. **Formaçâo profissional e inserçâo no mercado de trabalho** : perceptçoes de egressos de um curso de graduaçao em Enfermagem de instituiçao privada. 2009. 145 p.

Dissertaçao (Mestrado em enfermagem) - Universidade Estadual Paulista, Botucatu, 2009. Available at:

< http://repositorio.unesp.br/bitstream/handle/11449/96443/colenci_r_me_botfm.pdf?...1 >. Accessed: May 26, 2016.

COLENCI, Raquel; BERTI, Heloisa Wey. Formaçao profissional e inserçao no mercado de trabalho: percepçoes de egressos de graduaçao em enfermagem. **Revista da escola de enfermagem da USP** , Sao Paulo, v. 46, n. 1, p. 158-166, feb. 2012. Available at: < http://www.scielo.br/scielo.php?pid=S0080-62342012000100022&script=sci_arttext >. Accessed: May 26, 2016.

FEDERAL COUNCIL OF NURSING. **Resolution COFEN-293/2004** . Fixa e Estabelece Parametros para o Dimensionamento do Quadro de Profissionais de Enfermagem nas Unidades Assistenciais das Instituiçoes de Saùde e Assemelhados. Rio de Janeiro, September 21 . 2004. Available at: < http://www.cofen.gov.br/resoluo-cofen-2932004_4329.html >. Access em: 09 out. 2016.

REGIONAL NURSING COUNCIL. **Map da enfermagem de Santa Catarina** . Florianópolis, 2016. Available at: < http://www.corensc.gov.br/iframe/mapa_coren/ >.

Access em: 09 out. 2016.

DALLACOSTA, Fabiana Meneghetti; MAKOWSKI, Rosê Maria; TOMASI, Patricia Zilio. **Enfermagem na Unoesc Joaçaba** : 10 years of history. Joaçaba: Ed. Unoesc, 2016.

DELUIZ, Neise. Humanizar cuidados de saùde: uma questao de competencia. **Ministério da Saùde** , 2001. Available at: < http://bvsms.saude.gov.br/bvs/publicacoes/profae/Revista2002.pdf >. Accessed: 23 Jun 2016.

DIAS, Alexsandro de Oliveira; GUARIENTE, Maria Helena Dantas de Menezes; BELEI, Renata Aparecida. A recently graduated enfermeiro eo primeiro emprego. Percepçoes da formaçao na graduaçao e da atuaçao profissional. **Arquivos de Ciência da Saùde UNIPAR** , Umuarama, v. 8, n. 1, p. 19-24, Jan./Apr. 2004. Available at: < http://revistas.unipar.br/index.php/saude/article/view/237/210 >. Access em: 01 Jul. 2016.

FERREIRA, Rosa Gomes. Estresse do profissional de enfermagem no serviço noturno: uma questao de saùde. **Revista Saùde e Desenvolvimento** , v. 7, n. 4, Jan./Dec. 2015. Available at:

< http://www.grupouninter.com.br/revistasaude/index.php/saudeDesenvolvimento/article/view File/396/278 >. Access em: 06 out. 2016.

OSVALDO CRUZ FOUNDATION . **Pesquisa inèdita trace perfil da enfermagem no Brasil** . Rio de Janeiro, 2015. Available at: < http://portal.fiocruz.br/pt-br/content/pesquisa-inedita- traca-perfil-da-enfermagem-no-brasil >. Access em: 08 out. 2016.

IBGE. **Estimated population 2016** . Rio de Janeiro, 2016. Available at: < http://cidades.ibge.gov.br/xtras/perfil.php?lang=&codmun=420670&search=santa- catarina | herval-d'oeste >. Access em: 07 out. 2016.

JESUS, Bruna Helena de et al. Inserçao no mercado de trabalho: trajetória de egressos de um curso de graduaçao em enfermagem. **Escola Anna Nery** , Rio de Janeiro, v. 17, n. 2, p. 336 345, abr./jun. 2013. Available at: < http://www.scielo.br/pdf/ean/v17n2/v17n2a19.pdf >. Access em: 10 Aug. 2016.

JESUS, Elaine dos Santos et al. Preconceito na enfermagem: percepçao de enfermeiros formados em differentes decesas . **Revista da Escola de Enfermagem da USP** , Sao Paulo, v. 44, n. 1, p. 164-170. 2010. Available at: < http://www.revistas.usp.br/reeusp/article/download/40523/43617 >. Access em: 02 May. 2016.

JESUS, Bruna Helena de; GOMES, Diana Coelho; SPILERE, Lia Beatriz Bortolotto. **CONTRIBUIÇAO DA FORMAÇAO CRÌTICO - CRIATIVA NA INSERÇAO NO MERCADO DE TRABALHO: visâo de egressos de enfermagem** . Florianópolis, 2011. 88 p. Trabalho de Conclusao de Curso (Graduaçao em Enfermagem) - Universidade Federal de Santa Catarina, Florianópolis, 2011. Available at: < https://repositorio.ufsc.br/handle/123456789/121476 >. Access em: 19 out. 2016.

JUNGES, Kelen do Santos; BEHRENS, Marilda Aparecida. Pratica docente no Ensino Superior: a formaçao pedagogica como mobilizadora de muenda. **Respectiva** , Florianópolis, v. 33, n. 1, p. 285-317, Jan./Abr. 2015. Available at:

< https://periodicos.ufsc.br/index.php/perspectiva/article/view/2175-795X.2014v33n1p285/31220 >. Accessed: 02 May 2016.

LIMA, Càssio de Almeida; VIEIRA, Maria Aparecida; COSTA, Fernanda Marques yes. Caracterizaçao dos estudes do curso de graduaçao em Enfermagem de uma universidade pública. **Revista Norte Mineira de Enfermagem** , Monte Claros, v. 3, n. 2, p. 33-46. 2014. Available at: < http://www.renome.unimontes.br/index.php/renome/article/view/72/98 >. Access em: 07 out. 2016.

LIMA, Maria Alice Dias da Silva. Ensino de enfermagem: retrospective, current situation and perspective. **Revista Brasileira de Enfermagem** , Brasilia, v. 47, n. 3, p. 270-277, July/September. 1994. Available at: < http://www.scielo.br/scielo.php?script=sci_arttext&pid=S0034-71671994000300008 >. Access em: 14 out. 2016.

LIMA, Marlinir Bezerra de et al. Agentes stressores em trabajoles de enfermagem com dupla ou mais jornada de trabalho . **Research journal: Cuidado é fundamental online** , Rio de Janeiro, v. 5, n. 1, p. 3259-3266, Jan./Mar. 2016. Available at: < http://www.seer.unirio.br/index.php/cuidadofundamental/article/view/1907/pdf_683 >.

Access em: 12 out. 2016.

LOPES, Marta Julia Marques; LEAL, Sandra Maria Cezar. A persistent feminizaçao na qualificaçao profissionai da enfermagem brasileira. **Gènero e Saùde** , Porto Alegre, v. 24, p. 105-125, Jan./Jun. 2005. Available at: <http:// www.scielo.br/pdf/cpa/n24/n24a06.pdf >. Access em: 28 Aug. 2016.

LOPES, Lùcia Marlene Macàrio; SANTOS, Sandra Maria Pereira dos. Florence Nightingale - Apontamentos sobrea fundadora da Enfermagem Moderna. **Revista de Enfermagem Reference** , v. 3, n. 2, p. 181-189, dez. 2010. Available at: < http://www.scielo.mec.pt/pdf/ref/vserIIIn2/serIIIn2a19.pdf >. Access em: 25 Aug. 2016.

MACHADO, Maria Helena et al. Aspectos gerais da formationa da Enfermagem: o perfil da formationa dos Enfermeiros, Técnicos e Auxiliares. **Enfermagem em Foco** , v. 6, n. 2/4, p. 15 34, 2016. Available at: < http://revista.portalcofen.gov.br/index.php/enfermagem/article/view/687/297 >. Access em: 12 out. 2016 a.

MACHADO, Maria Helena et al. Mercado de trabalho da enfermagem: general aspects. **Enfermagem em Foco** , v. 6, n. 1/4, p. 43-78, 2016. Available at: < http://revista.portalcofen.gov.br/index.php/enfermagem/article/view/691 > . Access em: 07 out. 2016 b.

MAIA, Sayonara Ferreira. **Perfil dos egressos do curso de graduaçao em enfermagem de uma Universidade Federal** . 2014. 100 pp. Dissertaçao (Mestrado em Enfermagem)-Universidade Federal do Piaui, Teresina. Available at: < http://repositorio.ufpi.br/xmlui/handle/123456789/175 >. Accessed: 05 May 2016.

MAIER, Suellen Rodrigues de Oliveira; MATTOS, Magda de. O trabalhar eo estudiar no contexto universitàrio: uma approach com trabalhoder-estudantes. **Saùde** , Santa Maria, v. 42, n. 1, p. 179-185, Jan./Jun. 2016. Available at: < https://periodicos.ufsm.br/revistasaude/article/view/20477/pdf >. Access em: 12 out. 2016.

MALAGUTTI, Willian. Novas competencias na atuaçao dos enfermeiros no mundo globalizado. **J Management Primary Health Care** , Rio de Janeiro, v. 3, n. 2, p. 70-71, 2012. Available at: < www.jmphc.com.br/saude- publica/index.php/jmphc/article/download/140/142 >. Access em: 09 out. 2016.

MARTINS, Christiane et al. Enfermeiro profile and professional competence development needs . **Texto & Contexto - enfermagem** , Florianópolis, v. 15, n. 3, jun./set. 2006. Available at:

< http://www.scielo.br/scielo.php?script=sci_arttext&pid=S0104-07072006000300012 >. Access em: 20 Jul. 2016.

MATTOSINHO, Mariza Maria Serafim et al. Mundo do trabalho: alguns aspectso vivenciados pelos professionales néto-formados em enfermagem. **Acta Paulista de Enfermagem** , Sao Paulo, v. 23, n. 4, p. 466-471. 2010. Available at: < http://www.scielo.br/pdf/ape/v23n4/04.pdf >. Access em: 14 out. 2016.

MEDINA, Neuma Vital Julca ; TAKAHASHI, Queen Toshie . A busca da graduaçao em enfermagem como opçao dos técnicos e auxiliares de enfermagem. **Revista da Escola de Enfermagem da USP** , Sao Paulo, v. 37, n. 4, p. 101-108, 2003. Available at: < http://www.scielo.br/pdf/reeusp/v37n4/12.pdf >. Access em: 14 out. 2016.

MEIRA, Maria Dyrce Dias; KURCGANT, Paulina. Graduaçao segundo egressos evaluation course . **Revista da Escola de Enfermagem da USP** , Sao Paulo, v. 43, n. 2, p. 481-485, 2009. Available at: <http:// www.scielo.br/pdf/reeusp/v43n2/a31v43n2.pdf >. Access em: 10 set. 2016.

MORAIS, Marisa Pires de et al. Insatisfaçao no trabalho de enfermeiros de um

University Hospital. **Cogitare Enfermagem** , Paranà, v. 19, n. 2, p. 316-322, abr./jun. 2014. Available at: < http://revistas.ufpr.br/cogitare/article/view/31529/2275 >. Access em: 13 out. 2016.

MOREIRA, Augusto José do Nascimento et al. Mundo do trabalho: difficulties and challenges faced by newly admitted nurses in hospital units. **Revista Rede de Cuidados em Saùde** , Rio de Janeiro, v. 10, n. 3, p. 1-16, 2016. Available at: < http://publicacoes.unigranrio.br/index.php/rcs/article/view/3966/2047 >. Access em: 10 set. 2016.

NETO, José Milton Barros et al. A formaçao do profissional enfermeiro eo mercado de trabalho na actualidade. **Revista Eletrônica Gestao & Saùde** , v. 5, n. 1, p. 176-193. 2014. Available at: <

http://gestaoesaude.unb.br/index.php/gestaoesaude/article/view/675/pdf_1 >. Access em: 03 out. 2016.

NUNES, Carina Maria et al. Satisfaçao e insatisfaçao no trabalho na perceptçao de enfermeiros de um university hospital. **Revista Eletrônica de Enfermagem** , Goiânia, v. 12, n. 2, p. 252-257, abr./jun. 2010. Available at: < https://www.fen.ufg.br/fen_revista/v12/n2/v12n2a04.htm >. Access em: 05 out. 2016.

OLIVEIRA, Rafaela Bueno; TASHIMA, Cristiano Massao; COSTA, Talita Vidotte. Competências curriculares para a formaçao profissional: percepçao de enfermeiros egressos de uma Universidade Pùblica do Sul do Brasil. In: JORNADA DE INICIAÇÂO CIENTÌFICA DA UENP, 5., Bandeirantes. **Anais elektronikos** ... Paranà, 2015. Available at: <http://webcache.googleusercontent.com/search?q=cache:Mg25FPWedvsJ:www.uenp.edu.br/ certificados/propg/2015/Joic%2520V%2520 -

%2520UENP/Ciencias%2520da%2520Saude/RAFAELA%2520BUENO%2520OLIVEIRA.p df+&cd=1&hl=pt-BR&ct=clnk&gl=br>.

Access em: 04 out. 2016.

OLIVEIRA, Lilian Rodrigues et al. Trajetória profissional de egressos de enfermagem. **Interdisciplinar Magazine** , Teresina, v. 9, n. 1, p. 125-134, Jan./Mar. 2016. Available at: < http://revistainterdisciplinar.uninovafapi.edu.br/index.php/revinter/article/view/668/pdf_29 >. Access em: 10 Aug. 2016.

OGUISSO, Taka. **Trajetória histórica da enfermagem** . Barueri: Manole, 2014.

PAULA, Marcia Bernadete Leao dos Santos. **Inserçao do jovem no mercado de trabalho: as difficulties enfrentadas pelos jovens negros em busca do primeiro emprego** . 2012. 37 p. Monograph (Especializaçao em Gestao de Politicas Pùblicas com foco em Raça e Gênero)- Universidade Federal de Ouro preto, Conselheiro Lafaiete, 2012. Available at: < www.amde.ufop.br/tccs/Lafaiete/Lafaiete% 20-%20Marcia%20dos%20Santos.pdf > . Access em: 08 out. 2016.

PAVA, Andrea Macedo; NEVES, Eduardo Borba. A arte de ensarir enfermagem: uma história de sucesso. **Revista brasileira de enfermagem** , Brasilia, DF, v. 64, n. 1, Jan./Feb. 2011. Available at:

< http://www.scielo.br/scielo.php?script=sci_arttext&pid=S0034-71672011000100021 >. Access em: 23 set. 2016.

PEREIRA, Reinaldo Arruda. The importance of Scientific Initiation in academic formation and professional education. Davar **Policêmica magazine** , Belo Horizonte, v. 7, n. 1, p. 1-11, 2014.

Available at: http://sistemabatista.edu.br/SEER/index.php/DP/article/view/252/191 . Access em: 18 out. 2016.

PÜSCHEL, Vilanice Alves de Araùjo; INACIO, Mariana Pereira; PUCCI, Patricia Prici Agustini. Inserçao dos Egressos da Escola de Enfermagem da USP no Mercado de Trabalho: Facilidades e Dificuldades. **Revista da Escola de Enfermagem da USP** , Sao Paulo, v. 43, n. 3, p. 535-542, 2009. Available at: < http://www.producao.usp.br/handle/BDPI/4092 >.

Access em: 02 out. 2016.

RADIO CATARINENSE. **The State Governor inaugurates the expansion of HUST in Joaçaba** . Joaçaba, 2016. Available at:

< http://www.radiocatarinense.com.br/index.php/2016/04/08/governador-do-estado-inaugura-ampliacao-do-hust-em-joacaba/ >. Acesso em: 06 Nov. 2016.

RODRIGUES, Rosa Maria; CONTERNO, Solange by Fàtima Reis; GUEDES, Giovanna Carolina. Formaçao na graduaçao em enfermagem e impacto na atuaçao profissional na perspective de egressos. **Interfaces da Educaçao** , Paranaiba, v. 6, n. 17, p. 26-43, 2015.

Available at: < http://periodicosonline.uems.br/index.php/interfaces/article/view/744/685 >. Access em: 04 out. 2016.

ROVER, Ardinete; PEREIRA, Débora Diersmann Silva. **Diretrizes para elaboraçao de trabalhos cientificos** . Joaçaba UNOESC Publishing House, 2013.

SANTOS, Silvana Sidney Costa. Curriculos de enfermagem do Brasil e as directrizes - novas perspectivas. **Revista Brasileira de Enfermagem** , Brasilia, DF, v. 56, n. 4, p. 361-364, Jul./Aug. 2003. Available at: < http://www.scielo.br/pdf/reben/v56n4/a09v56n4.pdf >.

Access em: 17 Aug. 2016.

SILVA, Annyelle Magda Souza yes; OLIVEIRA, Mayara Evelin Soares de; OLIVEIRA, Rita Patricia Almeida de. Jovens Administradores eo Mercado de Trabalho. **Ciências humanas e sociais** , Recife, v. 2, n. 1, p. 39-52. 2015. Available at:

< https://periodicos.set.edu.br/index.php/facipehumanas/article/download/3052/1663 >. Access em: 15 out. 2016.

SILVA, Manoel Carlos Neri yes. Conselho Federa de Enfermagem no desenvolvimento de Politicas Pùblicas do Sistema Único de Saùde: Perspectivas e desafios. **Enfermagem em Foco** , v. 7, 2016. Available at: < http://revista.portalcofen.gov.br/index.php/enfermagem/article/view/698/308 >. Access em: 07 out. 2016.

SILVA, Mary Gome et al. Processo de formaçao da(o) enfermeira(o) na contemporaneidade: desafios e perspectivados. **Texto Contexto Enfermagem** , Florianópolis, v. 19, n. 1, p. 176-184, Jan./Mar. 2010. Available at: < http:// www.scielo.br/pdf/tce/v19n1/v19n1a21.pdf >. Access em: 01 out. 2016.

SOUZA, Ana Célia Caetano de et al. Formaçao do enfermeiro para o cuidado: reflexoes da pràtica professional. **Revista Brasileira de Enfermagem** , Brasilia, v. 59, n. 6 p. 805-807, Nov./Dec. 2006. Available at: < http://www.scielo.br/scielo.php?script=sci_arttext&pid=S0034-71672006000600016 >. Access em: 18 Aug. 2016.

SOUZA, Luis Paulo Souza et al. Os desafios da nête-formado em Enfermagem no mundo do trabalho. **Revista cubana de enfermagem** , v. 30, n. 1, 2014. Available at: < http://www.revenfermeria.sld.cu/index.php/enf/article/view/127/79 >. Access em: 16 set. 2016.

UNIVERSIDADE DO OESTE DE SANTA CATARINA. **Histórico** : Uma evoluçao perceived ao longo do tempo. Joaçaba, 2016. Available at: < http://www.unoesc.edu.br/unoesc/historico >. Access em: 08 out. 2016.

UNIVERSIDADE DO OESTE DE SANTA CATARINA. **University Project** . Fundaçao Educacional Unificada do Oeste de Santa Catarina. Porto Alegre: Evangelist, 1991.

UNIVERSIDADE DO OESTE DE SANTA CATARINA. **Pedagogical project of nursing course** . Joacaba, 2009.

VALL, Janaina; PEREIRA, Laura França; FRIESEN, Tatiane Temmy. O profil do acadêmico de Enfermagem em uma Privada Faculdade da cidade de Curitiba. **Cadernos da Escola de Saùde da UNIBRASIL** , Curitiba, v. 2, n. 1, p. 1-10, 2009. Available at:

< http://revistas.unibrasil.com.br/cadernossaude/index.php/saude/article/viewFile/18/18 >. Access em: 12 out. 2016.

APPENDIX A - SURVEY QUESTIONNAIRE

DATA COLLECTION FOR THE COURSE COMPLETION PROJECT

PROFILE OF UNOESC GRADUATES IN THE LABOR MARKET:

perceptions of training and professional activity

1 - What's your gender?

( ) Female ( ) Male

2 - How old are you?

3 - In which municipality do you live?

4 - In which municipality do you work?

5 - What year did you graduate?

---

6 - What was your occupation before studying nursing?

---

7 - Do you work as a nurse?

( ) Yes

( ) No

8 - What is your current occupation?

---

9 - Area of activity at the moment.

( ) Hospital

( ) Family Health Strategy

( ) Emergency Care Unit

( ) SAMU

( ) Teaching

( ) Clinics

( ) other

10 - How satisfied were you with the training you received during your degree?

( ) Full

( ) Partial

( ) Not much

( ) Did not

11 - What are your criticisms of your professional training?

---

12 - How would you rate your commitment to learning during the course?

( ) Full

( ) Partial

( ) Not much

( ) No commitment

13 - What difficulties did you face getting your first job as a nurse?

---

14 - How satisfied are you with your current professional activity?

( ) Very satisfied

( ) Satisfied

( ) Dissatisfied

( ) Very dissatisfied

15 - Have you done any of the specialties below?

( ) Specialization

( ) Master's degree

( ) Doctorate

( ) Other

( ) No courses

16 - How many jobs do you currently have as a nurse?

---

17 - What period do you work?

( ) Morning

( )Afternoon

( )Evening

( ) In two shifts

18 - What could have been improved during your degree course that you think would have helped you in your professional career and in the job market?

ANNEX A - OPINION OF THE RESEARCH ETHICS COMMITTEE

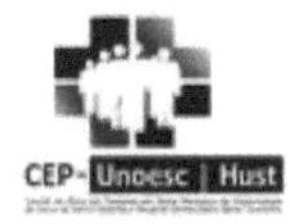

UNIVERSIDADE DO OESTE DE SANTA CATARINA - UNOESC

EXECUTIVE OPINION OF THE CEP

RESEARCH PROJECT DATA

Research Title: PROFILE **OF** UNOESC GRADUATES IN THE LABOR MARKET: Perceptions of training and professional performance

Researcher: Viviane koepp nardi

Thematic Area:

Version: 1

CAAE: 53978916.1.0000.5367

Proposing Institution: FUNDACAO UNIVERSIDADE DO OESTE DE SANTA CATARINA

Main Sponsor: Own Financing

OPINION DATA

Opinion Number: 1.482.384

Project presentation:

This is a research protocol for the preparation of a Course Conclusion Work, linked to the AREA OF LIFE SCIENCES of the Nursing Course at the Universidade do Oeste de Santa Catarina - Unoesc- Joaçaba, a research project authored by Renata Dalberto, under the supervision of Prof. Dr. Viviane Koepp Nardi.

Research Objective:

GENERAL OBJECTIVE

To characterize the profile and difficulties encountered by nurses after training and at the start of their professional careers.

SPECIFIC OBJECTIVES

Characterize the profile of nurses graduating from the UNOESC Joaçaba campus.

Analyze general and specific training, insertion in the job market and professional performance.

Describe the difficulties encountered in the academic-professional transition.

Endereço: Rua Getúlio Vargas, nº 2125, Centro Administrativo
Bairro: Flor da Serra **CEP:** 89.600-000
UF: SC **Município:** JOACABA
Telefone: (49)3551-2012 **Fax:** (49)3551-2004 **E-mail:** cep@unoesc.edu.br

Evaluation of Risks and Benefits:

Risks: Not applicable.

Benefits: Contributing to the university in terms of preparing graduates for the job market.

Comments and Considerations on the Research:

The presentation of the project is clear and objective, and concise, allowing us to conclude that the research proposal in question has a well-defined methodological approach, on the basis of which it will be possible to draw consistent and therefore valid conclusions.

It is recommended that the Conclusion item in the project be removed, as it is not applicable.

Considerations on Mandatory Terms of Presentation:

Presented in accordance with CNS/MS Resolution 466/12, the Rules of Procedure and Internal Regulations of the Research Ethics Committee, Universidade do Ceste de Santa Catarina - UNOESC.

* The Free and Informed Consent Form presented here complies with the provisions of CNS/MS Res. 466/12.
* Cover sheet o content meets specifications.
* Dispensation of the Term of Authorization for the Use of Images

Recommendations:

In accordance with Resolution 466/2015, it is recommended that researchers pay attention to the deadlines for submitting partial and final reports to this committee, and that they comply with the principle of beneficence by offering some form of feedback on the results to the research subjects.

We emphasize that the development of the research must follow the foundations, methodology, propositions, assumptions on screen, as they were presented and evaluated by this Research Ethics Committee. Any changes must be immediately reported to the CEP, via the Brazil Platform System, accompanied by the appropriate justifications:

1. An amendment is any proposed change to the original project, presented with the justification for it. Amendments must be presented to the CEP in a clear and succinct manner, identifying the part of the protocol to be modified and its justifications. The amendment will be analyzed by the following bodies

of its final approval (CEP and/or CONEP).

2. Extension is the proposal to extend or continue the research with the same recruited participants, without essential changes to the Objectives and methodology of the original project. If there are significant changes to the objectives and methods, another research protocol must be submitted. Researchers must observe and comply with the items listed below, as indicated by Res. 466/12:

a) develop the project as outlined;

b) prepare and present the final report;

c) submit data requested by CEP at any time;

d) keep your data in a physical or digital file for a period of 5 (five) years after the end of the research;

e) forward the results for publication, with due credit to the associated researchers and technical staff participating in the project;

f) justify the interruption of the project to CEP.

Conclusions or Pending Issues and List of Inadequacies:

In view of the APPROVAL opinion, there are no pending issues to be resolved in the research protocol.

The research protocol is considered completed.

Final considerations at the discretion of the REC:

This opinion was drawn up on the basis of the documents listed below:

Document Type	Archive	Post	Author	Situation
Basic Project	PB_BASIC_INFORMATION	26/02/2016		Accepted
Detailed Project / Investor Brochure	Project.doc	26/02/2016 17:42:28	Viviane koepp nardi	Accepted
Cover Sheet	folharosto.docx	26/02/2016	Viviane koepp nardi	Accepted
Others	formulariodeencaminhamento.doc	26/02/2016	viviane koepp nardi	Accepted
Others	Research project.doc	26/02/2016	Viviane koepp nardi	Accepted
TCLE / Terms of	Free_Consent_Form	26/02/2016	viviane koepp nardi	Accepted

Endereço: Rua Getúlio Vargas, nº 2125, Centro Administrativo
Bairro: Flor da Serra **CEP:** 89.600-000
UF: SC **Município:** JOACABA
Telefone: (49)3551-2012 **Fax:** (49)3551-2004 **E-mail:** cep@unoesc.edu.br

Assent / Reason for Absence	clarified.doc	09:49:21	Viviane koepp nardi	Accepted

Status of the opinion:

Approved

Needs CONEP appraisal:

No

JOACABA, April 07, 2016

Signed by:
Marcio Giusti Trevisol
(Coordinator)

Endereço: Rua Getúlio Vargas, nº 2125, Centro Administrativo
Bairro: Flor da Serra **CEP:** 89.600-000
UF: SC **Município:** JOACABA
Telefone: (49)3551-2012 **Fax:** (49)3551-2004 **E-mail:** cep@unoesc.edu.br

ANNEX B - INFORMED CONSENT FORM

INFORMED CONSENT FORM

You are being invited as a volunteer to take part in the research: **Profile of nursing graduates in the world of work: from training to professional activity**.

BACKGROUND, OBJECTIVES AND PROCEDURES: The reason for proposing this study is to get to know the profile of nursing graduates from UNOESC, Joaçaba campus, in order to help improve the quality of academic training and to identify the difficulties encountered by students working at the university when entering the job market. The research is justified by the fact that there are few studies on the subject, and there are none at UNOESC, as well as the importance of knowing the profile of graduates and their academic - professional transition. The aim of this project is to characterize the profile and difficulties encountered by nurses in the academic-professional transition.

The data collection procedure(s) will be as follows: A questionnaire will be sent electronically (Google Docs) containing 17 open and closed questions on: identification data, general and specific training, professional insertion and performance, with a deadline of two months for return. The data obtained will then be tabulated in Excel and converted into tables and graphs. The open questions will be described in full for the paper.

DISCOUNTS, RISKS AND BENEFITS: There will be no discomforts or risks since this is a research proposal using a questionnaire containing open and closed questions by electronic means. Your participation in this study will contribute to characterizing the profile of nurses graduating from the UNOESC Joaçaba campus, analyzing general and specific training, insertion in the job market and professional performance and describing the difficulties encountered in the academic-professional transition, contributing to improvements in teaching that can contribute to insertion and performance in the professional market.

GUARANTEE OF DISCLOSURE, FREEDOM OF REFUSAL AND GUARANTEE OF SECILITY: You may ask for clarification about the research at any stage of the study. You are free to refuse to take part, withdraw your consent or stop taking part in the study at any time, whether for reasons of embarrassment or otherwise. Your participation is voluntary and refusal to participate will not result in any penalty or loss of benefits. The researcher(s) will treat your identity with professional standards of confidentiality. The results of the research will be sent to you and will remain confidential. Your name or material indicating your participation will not be released without your permission. You will not be identified in any publication that may result from this study. This consent form is printed and signed in two copies, one copy will be given to you and the other will be kept by the researcher(s) responsible.

PARTICIPATION COSTS, REIMBURSEMENT AND INDEMNIFICATION: Participation in the study will not entail any costs for the participant and no financial compensation will be provided. If you suffer any damage as a result of this research, please contact the person responsible for the research or the student at the following address.

DECLARATION BY THE PARTICIPATING SUBJECT OR THE PERSON RESPONSIBLE FOR THE PARTICIPATING SUBJECT

I was

informed of the objectives of the above research in a clear and detailed manner and clarified my doubts. I know that I can ask for further information or withdraw my consent at any time. Those responsible for the above research have assured me that all my data will be kept confidential. If I have any questions, I can call the student Renata Dalberto, residing at Avenida Airton Senna da Silva, n° 659, casa 3, bairro Jardim Alvorada in the municipality of Joaçaba - SC, telephone contact: (49) 9961-6758 and the researcher in charge Viviane Koepp Nardi, 2521-2071, or contact the Ethics Committee for Research in Human Beings at Unoesc and Hust, Rua Getúlio Vargas, n° 2125, Bairro Flôr da Serra, 89600-000- Joaçaba - SC, Phone: 49-3551-2012. I declare that I agree to take part in this study. I have received a copy of this informed consent form and have been given the opportunity to read it and clarify my doubts.

Signature of the research subject or **fingerprint**.

Signature:

Legible name: Address: ID.

Phone:

Date // ____

Fingerprinting

Signature of the researcher responsible

Date // ____

ANNEX C - EMAIL INTERVIEW

De : Renata Dalberto <rd.jba@hemosc.org.br> Ter, 04 de Out de 2016 15:23
Assunto : Pesquisa 1 anexo
Para : leandracancian@yahoo.com.br

Boa tarde

Cara Leandra!

Venho por meio deste solicitar uma informação para fundamentar meu Trabalho de Conclusão de Curso. Preciso saber quantos enfermeiros estão atuando no HUST, pois meu indicador demonstrou que a maioria dos egressos da UNOESC atuam em Joaçaba.

Aguardo

Desde já, agradeço

Atenciosamente

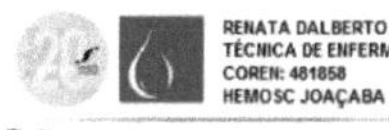

Antes de imprimir esta mensagem pense em sua responsabilidade e compromisso com o meio ambiente.

De : leandra del pizzol cancian <leandracancian@yahoo.com.br> Ter, 04 de Out de 2016 15:29
Assunto : Re: Pesquisa 1 anexo
Para : Renata Dalberto <rd.jba@hemosc.org.br>
Responder para : leandra del pizzol cancian <leandracancian@yahoo.com.br>

Olá!

Enfermeiros 64

Att.

Leandra Cancian
COREN SC 126628 Enf
Coordenadora da Equipe de Enfermagem HUST

De : Renata Dalberto <rd.jba@hemosc.org.br> Ter, 04 de Out de 2016 16:51
Assunto : Re: Pesquisa 2 anexos
Para : leandra del pizzol cancian <leandracancian@yahoo.com.br>

Obrigada

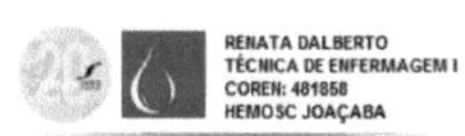

Antes de imprimir esta mensagem pense em sua responsabilidade e compromisso com o meio ambiente.

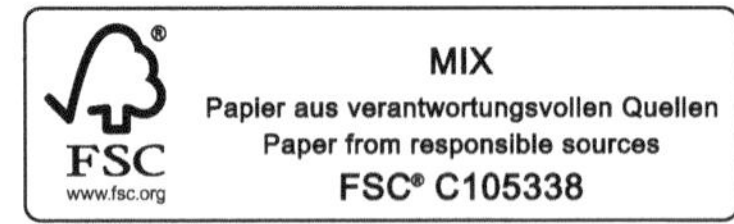

Printed by Books on Demand GmbH, Norderstedt / Germany